What's In Your 24?

How To
Get It Done
Without
Getting
Outdone

Dana Simone Stovall

outskirts press

Outskirts Press, Inc.
http://www.outskirtspress.com

Paperback ISBN: 978-1-4787-1177-3
Hardback ISBN: 978-1-4787-1142-1

Library of Congress Control Number: 2013902955

Outskirts Press and the "OP" logo are trademarks belonging to Outskirts Press, Inc.

PRINTED IN THE UNITED STATES OF AMERICA

ACKNOWLEDGEMENTS

First and foremost, thank you, Heavenly Father, for the gift of life. You have shown me so much favor and mercy, and I am forever grateful.

Destiny, I can only hope and pray that I have been the best mother you could ever wish for. Since you were born, you've taught me so much about life, sacrifice, endurance, happiness, and unconditional love. You make me so proud, Angel Girl, and I love you with all my heart.

Mom, Billy, Grandma Florence, and JoAnne, our family may be small, but the love, support, and joy that you've always shown me are immeasurable. Although there are many miles, mountains, and molehills between our zip codes, nothing stands in the way of our unity. I love you wholeheartedly!

Angela, Carol, Derek, Krystal, Micheal, LaShanda, all of my many friends, mentors, mentorees, other "moms and dads," and pastors that I dare not attempt to name them all specifically, thank you for trusting me, encouraging me, and telling me what I needed to hear, not what I wanted to hear. I sincerely appreciate you being a part of my "village"!

Nina Rawls, host of the 2day2nite Show, thank you for the rare opportunity to co-host with you and George. Your show was 1st to discuss my book and I sincerely appreciate it very much! Let's have a bonfire in Arizona soon. O-H…I-O!! Smooches

Miguel Calhoun, Bill Hill, and Rondi Stickney, you are the best health and fitness trainers in the Midwest. Thank you for your hard-core techniques to keep this old woman in shape!

Ladies from the Living Life Without Excuses group, thank you for trusting me and being the first to test the effectiveness of my Time Efficiency Tips™! You all rock: Angela V, Bernadette D, Brenda F, Carmesha S, Carol B, Chiquita W, Cierra W, Catherine J, Danielle B, Deanne K, Debra F, Denise M, Donna B, Dora B, Dorothy A, Forestine B, Glenda H, Emma R, Ivy M, Janine B, June C, Kathleen S, Keetie J, Kendra M, Kenya K, Kim B, LaTonya B, LaShanda T, Laura P, Lisa R, Michelamonie W, Nena T, Nicole S, Pamela C, Regina W, Renee M, Shalita W, Tamara H, Teri C, Theresa A, Tiffany H, Toni F, Valeria H, Valerie A, Veda G, and Veronica S.

TABLE OF CONTENTS

Rise and Shine

How many times have you said, "I wish I had more hours in a day," "I need time for me," or "Where did the time go?" You say these things because you don't feel you have enough time to do the things you need or want to do. However, the problem is not the *amount* of time you have; it's how you choose to *use* that time.

It seems like no matter how many attempts you make to get things done, you never seem to conquer that evil To Do List. Whether it's inclement weather, your children's activities, your spouse's list, extended family drama, health issues, or just plain lack of desire, that list is never completed.

English Chambers Dictionary defines time as the continuous passing and succession of minutes, days, and years. The operative word here is *continuous.* Time continues to pass, and what do we do? We continue to take advantage of those minutes, days, and years.

The contents of this book will attempt to squash the misnomer that is common in every-day language: *I don't have time.* Begin to think of it this way: when we are blessed to breathe another day, we all start with the same 24 hours. I have never met anyone who said that a full day equals 15 or 20 hours. So when someone asks us, "Did you exercise today?" or "Did you call your best friend last night?" why do we respond by saying, "I didn't have time"? As we all know, 1 day consists of 24 hours, and that's not going to change. However, what we can change are the choices we make to use those hours each day.

This book is for moms, married, divorced, single women, and even widows who desire a practical guide that speaks to their specific needs and helps them maximize their 24 more efficiently and effectively.

I realize there are hundreds of How-To and Self-Help books and other resources that dis-cuss time management with the use of handy notebooks and leather planners. You've even seen people in their car at the traffic light mov-ing their lips purposefully, and when you stare carefully, they are chanting along with their self-help CD yelling, "I am wonderful—I am beautiful." Seriously?! Not quite the motivation I need, what about you?

Don't get me wrong or send me a nasty gram, because some planners are good resources for many people; but oftentimes, you need a week or 2 and sometimes a video tutorial just to learn how to use it. And you're probably saying to yourself right now, "I don't have time for that."

I like to affectionately categorize those books as "shelf-help," because you read it once and put it on a shelf. Then what? You probably don't change. What happens is that you make temporary modifications to your behavior, then after a little while, revert back to what was comfortable.

I'm not prophesying that once you read 24 you will jump into a phone booth and fly out of it transformed with a Superwoman cape to boot. But I want 24 to get you thinking about a personal lifestyle change, and the distinct difference between a typical "shelf-help" book and 24.

One difference about 24 is that it will assist in holding you accountable for the covenants you make with yourself. Then we'll work on that phone booth and cape. Another difference about *24* from a typical "shelf-help" is that when you complete the book, I want you to stay in contact with me to keep me informed of your progress. I'm here to reassure you that you are not alone in your quest for reaching the ultimate level of abundant living and being honestly happy.

What's the point of reading *24* if you don't have a support system of other women to bounce ideas and strategies off of during your lifestyle changes, to get encouragement from success stories, or just to brag to someone who really gives a damn? (Oooh, pray church!)

I emphasize that last point because have you ever noticed when you make fabulous fitness and health choices, people start hating on you? People say things like, "Why do you work out so much . . .?" "Don't worry about that muffin; one muffin won't kill you . . ." "You are crazy for eating that organic mess . . ." "That's all you are going to eat . . .?" "Girl, I can't be bothered with all that . . ." Or, "Ain't nobody got time for that."

People say these things because they feel they have the right to judge you. They are envious of your dedication and commitment. Some don't want to see you happy. Many people are simply ignorant of what health and fitness are really about.

24 contains three chapters. Yes, that's it—three. Remember the Jackson 5's lyrics "It's easy as 1, 2, 3"? Well, this is my attempt at easy. The chapters are Vision, Brain Surgery, and Application. We all have visions of something that we desire to do. But ask yourself how long you've had this vision and what have you done to implement it.

Implementing a vision is to apply the objectives thereof. Whether that's opening a business, finding another job, going back to college, or losing weight. The only way to achieve your goals is by assassinating your inner voice that screams negativity and slowly suffocates your self-esteem.

If you took 10 percent of the energy you put into other people's agendas and applied that to your own goals, we could all be healthy, happy, and fit Superwomen.

Brain Surgery discusses the importance of

programming your mind to do what you envision doing; to do things you always wanted to do for yourself.

Brain Surgery is also the most important part of *24*, because the highway to changing your lifestyle begins with your mind, the most powerful asset you own and control. Once you can perform that delicate yet necessary surgery of replacing excuses with motivators, life becomes easier and less complicated.

Application focuses on the second-most important part of this book: applying what you've learned. We've all heard the phrase: knowledge is power. Well, I learned years ago from one of my favorite motivational speakers, Jonathan Sprinkles, that knowledge really isn't power. *Applied* knowledge is power.

I've come to realize since he made that statement that if you never apply what you learn, then you are merely a library. As you know, a library contains millions of books and resources, but if no one ever used them, the library merely takes up land and space.

Application is also my favorite chapter, because it provides everyday examples of what I've coined as Time Efficiency Tips™ (TETs). TETs are those practical things I've learned and done through the years to stay in control and become a happier Superwoman with the cape. You can use TETs right now without the fancy note-books, planners, and video instructions. These TETs are simple, raw, and for women who want to get it done without getting *out*done. TETs make it hard for anyone to make excuses for not doing them because they fit so well within the course of everything you do every day.

My friends, *24* is the book you've all been wait-ing for. It's the first edition of the lifestyle bible. *24* is the guide to living happier, getting fit from the inside out, taking control of your destiny, and living life without excuses. *24* will empower you, make you laugh, and make you cry. But most im-portantly, *24* will make you take a long look at yourself and help you determine why you aren't living a life of Ephesians 3:16.

When you're done reading *24*, you will learn how to love you more, how to prioritize your thoughts and efforts, how to quiet the chat-ter around you and think clearer, and how to exercise at least three times a day without much effort. Above all, you'll learn how to walk with a smile and put a pep in your step that reflects confidence, strength, high self-esteem, and a glow that stops people in their tracks to take a double look at you.

Now, what I don't want 24 to be is a thick "shelf-help" book with hundreds of pages for you to sort through just to get the point.

One of the things I learned while working at McDonald's Corporation on an executive leadership project was "Be Bright * Be Brief * Be Gone." This slogan was on a desk trinket that I immediately took to heart and applied in my daily living. That's why I formatted 24 to be concise, pocket-sized, and a very easy read. I want to inspire and motivate you to change your life right now, and it shouldn't take 2 or 3 weeks for me to do that.

Shouldn't a guide about time efficiency be efficient with your time?

This book has 12 sections to emulate the 12 hours on a clock. Also, there are 24 TETs to remind you that you have the same 24 hours as the next person to get things done.

Finally, I've intentionally written 24 on 60

pages. It's my desire that this book shouldn't take you more than 60 minutes to read it, more than 60 seconds to make the decision to change your life, and no more than 24 hours to begin making that transformation.

Tick Tock ⏱

CHAPTER 1

Vision

. . . Where there is no vision, the people will perish (Proverbs 29:18).

Who are you? Can you answer that question with no hesitation? If you take a minute and think back 5, 10, or 25 years ago, what did you say you wanted to be when you grew up? A doctor, politician, an actress, wife, mother, business owner? Now, look in the mirror and tell me what you see. If you don't see that image in the mirror, you are going to love this chapter!

I believe vision is the foundation of our existence. It's one of those precious gifts from God that some either fail to recognize or fail to fully utilize. Keep in mind, vision is not discriminatory; it resonates within all of us. Once you recognize your vision, your purpose in life becomes Swarovski clear. But you must give yourself a little credit for being as brilliant as you are and act on that vision.

One O'clock: Put Action in Your Vision

Once you have developed a vision, set a goal. Every goal requires objectives or implementation steps. For example, to make a cake is a goal. Purchasing the ingredients, preparing your cooking area, and mixing the ingredients are essential steps to make that cake.

Let me share a personal story about one of my visions that I transformed into a goal. In August 1988, 2 months after I turned 18 years old, I ventured away from my Detroit home to attend Wiley College in Marshall, Texas . . . Home of the Great Debaters. That fall semester, the college hosted a career fair.

At the time, I was exploring the possibility of becoming a stockbroker, but I had not narrowed down my ideal career just yet. As I walked around to the different company tables, I listened to the company pitches about their positions and benefits. Then I approached a table with a sign that read: FDIC. My only vague recollection of the FDIC was merely the black and gold signs I noticed when I, as a child, accompanied my dad to Comerica Bank. So I stopped, and the recruiter began to tell me about the FDIC and its Outstanding Scholar Program. The recruiter stated that the FDIC was a federal government agency under the Department of the Treasury with great benefits, stability, vast promotional opportunities, and a rewarding career in public service. He added that if I maintained a 3.45 GPA in a business-related major with 6 hours in accounting, I could be hired by the FDIC with no hoops to jump through when I graduated.

I thought to myself, *That's easy; I can do that.* I knew I wanted a stable career that would be flexible enough to allow me to pursue my other passions and that provided great benefits and salary potential (the entry level salary of $23,997 didn't sound like much at the time, though).

I got stability and longevity insight from my mom, who retired from a telephone company, and my dad, who retired from the United States Postal Service. Both of my parents had stable jobs with great benefits so I always knew I would choose a career with the same qualities.

On that day of the career fair, I decided that I would become a bank examiner with the FDIC. It became motivation for me to keep my GPA high so I would qualify for the job in 4 years.

Four years?! Yes, 4 years! Why not? I was

informed of a great stable company with a powerful mission, excellent benefits, and the qualifications I needed to apply. Therefore, it became my vision at 18 years old to work for the FDIC.

Then, I determined that I needed a plan to accomplish my goal by directing all of my academic energy into becoming an outstanding scholar at Wiley College. For the next 4 years, I made all As and Bs (never got a C). Well, let me say that I was lucky not to have Dr. "I Give You F" Clayton as one of my professors. I developed leadership skills by maintaining numerous officer roles in campus organizations, such as UNCF's Pre-Alumni Council, class president, and class treasurer.

Almost every year, the FDIC visited the campus for career day, and I stopped by their table to talk with the recruiter. If the initial recruiter I met in 1988 didn't attend, the current recruiter was told about me in advance and was advised to check out my transcript to make sure I was still on track for potential employment.

In April 1992, 1 month before graduation, I contacted FDIC for an application. In May, I graduated magna cum laude. In June, I interviewed with FDIC in Dallas, Texas. In July, I was hired as an assistant bank examiner with the FDIC.

Two O'clock: Never Negotiate Nonnegotiables

Notice, I never referenced that I interviewed with several companies in June. I never even called or sought after another company besides the FDIC. I already had the vision when I was a freshman, developed into a leader and outstanding scholar, and completed the qualifications, so there was no need to negotiate that vision.

Wow, what a vision, right? Many of you may ask me, was it easy? As Whitney Houston would say, "Hell to the naw." My college years were extremely difficult and very painful. I encountered numerous distractions. Heck, I think I had more fights and curve balls in college than I did in my entire childhood. Distractions such as fighting one of my roommates and my sorority line sisters, such as trashing clothes that people ripped in my closet while I was out of town on school business, and such as dating the loser boyfriend. But through it all, I focused on the goals. I kept my long-term desires at the forefront of my mind like a pot of gold at the end of the rainbow.

Besides my parents' strict influence and the thought of making them proud, grace and determination enabled me to focus and conquer my distractions at such a formative age.

I was also of the mind-set that I didn't have to personally experience tragedy and devastation in order to learn many of life's lessons. If I saw tragedy happen to someone else, I believed it could happen to me. I quickly learned from other people's mistakes to avoid repeating history.

So, there it is! Almost 21 years later, I have a great career, and I love it! That, my friends, is Vision at its best!

Three O'clock: Filter Your Thoughts

Let me spend a moment discussing how you filter your thoughts to select a vision that is about you and directly benefits you. I am not speaking of the visions you have that involve your children, spouse, or friends. Remember, this book is for the transformation of you.

In light of the fact that you have so many visions and dreams, you have to determine which visions to foster. It's not realistic to think that you can accomplish all of your hopes and dreams within your lifetime, because like most people, you probably have a "bucket list" longer than a mile. The key is to pick those dreams that will give you long-term happiness, a feeling of self-worth, and a stable life foundation.

While happiness and self-worth require no explanation, a stable life foundation is living a life that can withstand most obstacles you might encounter with minimal disruption to your day-to-day agenda or lifestyle.

In order to guarantee such a firm foundation, you must always make today's choices based upon tomorrow's unknowns.

That doesn't mean dwell on all the negative "what-ifs" until you talk yourself out of doing something, but it means to give consideration to anything that may derail your plan and to develop backup solutions that will keep you on the right track.

Finally, don't be so stubborn or inflexible to see a bigger picture and modify your actions accordingly. Oftentimes, we look at something and think we see exactly what's there, but if we back up a few steps, we can see a totally different image from a broader perspective.

I was watching a movie a few years ago that

included a segment about a photographer who was taking pictures for hours somewhere in a tropical area trying to get the best shot for a magazine story. After several rolls of film, he climbed to the top of a mountain and directly across from him he spotted a beautiful flower that bloomed along the side of that mountain. He immediately focused in on that flower and took many shots of it, perfectly angled and polarized color.

All of a sudden, something told him to zoom his lens out. What he saw was amazing! It was the picture he was looking for. Surrounding what he thought was a perfect vision of a blooming flower was a waterfall. The waterfall was calm yet rapid enough that the water flow created a mist that appeared as if magical clouds were protecting the flower.

The photographer described that moment as putting yourself in a position to achieve the greatest potential. That was the broader perspective. If the photographer had never stepped back to see the bigger picture, he would have missed that opportunity of capturing the perfect image.

We all have many things we want to accomplish in life, but it's important to know which goals will help us achieve the greatest potential; in other words, bear the most fruit. When I say "fruit," I'm not necessarily inferring money, because money is not as sustainable as becoming a well-rounded, diverse, and highly skilled woman. I like to call this creating a female masterpiece.

Four O'clock: The Female Masterpiece

The female masterpiece is a woman fully equipped with the necessary armor, knowledge, skills, and abilities to transform herself when she has to, and more importantly, when she *wants* to.

I strongly believe that one of the reasons that many women say, "I gave him all of me and now I don't know who I am" after a divorce or stay in abusive relationships is because too many women fail to remain true to their identity once they get married or have children. No one should expect you to change who you are at any point in your life, whether you are single or married. If you are in college, stay in college until you graduate. If you were working before you got married, continue to work. This economy proves to be unpredictable, and no matter how much money you think your spouse provides today, tomorrow's wealth isn't promised.

If you have any skills or abilities that can earn you money or that will allow you to maintain a competitive edge in the workplace, keep nurturing them. Don't lose sight of the blind spots. Always have a Plan B, because A could malfunction at any time.

The best way I explain this to women that confide in me is that I ask them 2 similar questions. *What are you capable of doing if your spouse was not around?* I mean, if one day you kissed your spouse good-bye in the morning and he or she was hit and killed in a car accident that afternoon. After all the relatives and friends go back to their respective lives and the kids are back in school, do you have the ability to maintain your current lifestyle and support your family?

Now, think about the more common occurrence: a divorce. If you and your spouse divorced today, after all the court papers are finalized, after you've cried your eyeballs out, and after you've eaten all the bonbons, *do you have what it takes by yourself to maintain your standard of living that you've become accustomed to?*

Most women I've talk to answer those questions with a resounding *no.*

Here's where becoming a female masterpiece comes into play. If you aren't that masterpiece right now, begin your metamorphosis. Start reading *USA Today* and watching CNN to keep a cursory knowledge of what's going on in the world and how that might affect you, directly or indirectly. Regardless of how it might affect you, brace yourself.

Here's a simple example. When I heard on the news that the Apple iPhone was coming out, I devised a plan to get that phone. The news came out in January, and the phone was being released in June of that same year. I determined how many paychecks I would receive between January and June, then I divided the number of checks by the cost of the phone. I then set up an automatic transfer of that amount from my checking account to my highest interest-bearing account every 2 weeks. By the time the phone was released, I had the funds to purchase it, plus I earned a little interest in the process.

I use this strategy for most of my financial decisions. Believe it or not, I never pay the full amount of a bill from a single paycheck.

Stretching my dollar over a period of time keeps me from taking several hundred dollars from one check, or even worse, getting a credit card to pay for something. E-mail me if you want to know the details of my dollar-stretching concept.

Five O'clock: Get Out of Bedrock

Guess what? Technology isn't going anywhere. Stop being afraid and start developing the necessary skills. If you can't operate the basic retail or corporate computers and software, you are significantly stifling your income potential. You can't expect to get a job or keep a job if you become more extinct than a typewriter.

You can't continue to use your generational title as an excuse. Whether you're a baby boomer, traditionalist, or Generation X, you must remain relevant.

When I attended Wiley College, I didn't own a fancy laptop or any type of computer, so when I graduated and started at FDIC, I had to force myself to learn how to use the equipment and software.

The first day on the job, they gave me a laptop

with all the latest software, a 10-key adding machine, and an Hp financial calculator. I was thinking, *seriously?!* But I learned them. They came with tutorials and user guides that became my best friends. It was not long before I started to become very proficient at using all of it. My performance evaluations never slammed me for not being familiar with the technology.

You know what happens when you aren't a female masterpiece—somebody else controls some part of you. I don't know about you, but I like being in control at all times. Or at least God lets me believe that I am.

By the way, men aren't that fond of all the parts of a female masterpiece, so you have to learn how to let them think they are running things. If a man suspects that you don't need him for anything, chances are eventually he may not consider the relationship fulfilling. And you might end up eternally single like me, so ladies, don't go overboard.

The application process within many of the federal agencies is built around whether the applicant has the basic knowledge, skills, and abilities (KSAs) to qualify for a position.

If you think about it from a practical standpoint, KSAs are the basic foundation that everyone should spend a large portion of their life enhancing.

I've learned that no matter what your occupation or interests are, personally or professionally, it's paramount to remain relevant and competitive with strong KSAs.

A couple of years ago when I was selected to participate in a leadership program called the Executive Potential Program offered at the FDIC, I read a book titled *Off-Ramps and On-Ramps, Keeping Talented Women on the Road to Success*, by Sylvia Hewlett. During Hewlett's 35-year career, she experienced changes in her career pattern such as working full-time, part-time, and not working at all due to her personal responsibilities, including motherhood. She coined these working patterns "off-ramps," "on-ramps," and "scenic routes."

One of the things that became apparent to me was that women who off-ramped, then on-ramped, had the KSAs to do so. Why? Because they remained relevant during the time that they took maternity leave or any extended amount of leave.

The male-dominated career model has no sympathy for women without the necessary skill set to do the job "they" want you to do.

Now, think about what you want to be when you grow up. Something you want to do. Somewhere you want to go. Take that vision, develop a plan, and live every day fanatical about implementing that plan. It really is that simple.

Tick Tock ⏲

CHAPTER 2

Brain Surgery

*. . . Do not conform any longer to the pat-
tern of this world, but be transformed by
the renewal of your mind (Romans 12:2).*

M y friends, this is the most important
chapter of this book! When I began writing this chapter I told myself, *"Self, the readers
are not going to like what I have to say here."* But
what I'm about to point out will clarify why we
don't get things done.

Unfortunately, sometimes we have to hear
things we don't want to hear. For instance, we've
all seen that female at the nightclub or restaurant with her friends, and she looks a hot mess.
Her outfit is too small, her boobs are too big for
the shirt, her hair is off da' hook, or she has on
too much makeup.

Then your mind quickly assesses the sit-
uation and you say to yourself, *"Self, that
female over there has two problems. She doesn't*

have mirrors in her house, and she needs new friends."

For argument's sake, her friends probably picked her up from her house and allowed her to walk out in public looking like that without saying one word to her. You see my point?

Ladies, you have to be a real friend and point those little things out to help nurture your friendships and save you and your buddies some embarrassment.

Now, don't be offended or throw the book away after you read this chapter. I'm merely pointing out, as a friend (smile), some things that somebody should have told you, like I wish they would have told me, a long time ago.

Six O'clock: Poison Ivy

One of the reasons we don't get things done or do what we dream of doing is because we have poisoned our minds to believe that everyone else is more important than ourselves.

If you've ever seen an episode of Oprah regarding women who are unhappily married or you've listened to one of your girlfriends complain about her life, the first thing they say is "I don't know who I am anymore" or "Everything I did in my life was for my husband and children."

The problem is that before women enter their marriage, they forget to set the groundwork for eternal marital bliss, which is making sure your significant other understands that he is *not* the most important person in your life, but that *you* are. Which means that you will take care of you first and everybody else is secondary, and under no condition is that ever negotiable.

The matter in which you start a relationship with your mate is usually how it will play out through its duration. That is why your happiness should be the first and most important vision you have and achieve.

Seven O'clock: If Momma Ain't Happy

We've all heard the saying that if momma ain't happy, ain't nobody happy. The people affected by your unhappiness usually include your kids, spouse, partner, significant other, friends, coworkers, and anyone else you have direct contact with. You might be thinking that's a little dramatic but let's analyze it further.

When I speak about happy, I mean it in the

literal sense in that happy is your attitude. For example, if you're not feeling well, you may not want to cook a large meal like you normally do, so beans and franks become the gourmet spread for that particular day. Thus, the affected people are your family, who always look forward to your "June Cleaver" meals.

Another example is if you wake up on the wrong side of the bed, traffic is heavier than usual, and the kids are fighting in the car again. By the time you arrive at work (three minutes shy of a meeting presentation), your nerves are shot, and you're completely irritated. The affected people are everyone in attendance at your meeting. Instead of hearing from an intelligent, well-versed, and dynamic speaker, they get the "let me get this over with so I can go to my office" speaker.

Do you see the point I'm making? Happy is truly your frame of mind. In order to achieve ultimate control of your happiness, you have to program your mind or perform mental Brain Surgery by convincing yourself that it's not about everybody else, but that it's all about you—first.

I see people spend their entire week running their kids around, making their spouse's lunch, paying the bills, and serving on all the church committees, but rarely do they take time for themselves to go to the fitness center or get a massage.

Eight O'clock: Learn to Be a Little Selfish

Ladies, you have to learn how to love yourself a lot more and cater to everyone else a little less. In essence, be more selfish with how you allow others to manipulate your time.

Yes, I said, selfish!

Encarta World English Dictionary states that "selfish" means two things: (1) concerned with your own interests, needs, and wishes while ignoring those of others and (2) showing that personal needs and wishes are thought to be more important than those of other people.

Both definitions basically reference concern with one's own needs and wishes, but I view them with a clear, distinct difference.

Like the Holy Bible, everyone interprets it differently, and so here's my interpretation of selfish.

Selfish definition (1) is beneficial for you, but not for your family and friends, because while you are busy taking care of you, you also ignore everyone else and fail to foster other's happiness.

However, Selfish definition (2) is beneficial for everyone around you, because you take care of yourself first, and then everyone else. It doesn't state that you ignore the needs of others like Selfish (1). To me, Selfish (2) implies your needs come first; and there is absolutely nothing wrong with that.

Do the things you NEED to do for yourself, then do what you WANT to do for others. Understand the difference. Doing for you is not a want; it's a need. And being selfish is OK if your core of concerns and needs include your mate, children, friends, and community; but only if you take care of you first.

I am all about making other people feel happy and secure, but never by sacrificing me like a lamb in the process.

How many of you just reread the last two sentences and your eyebrow peaked on the word "community"? Let me explain.

One of the reasons we should pursue true happiness is so that we can do a better job of being Christians or spiritual servants in our community.

Have you ever noticed that the majority of

people that spend a lot of time, money, or put effort into community service are those who appear to be honestly happy? That's because people who are happy and self-confident feel a sense of obligation to help others achieve that same feeling and empowerment. Besides, have you ever seen a severely depressed person giving their time or sharing their skills to empower others? Probably not.

Nine O'clock: Insanity

Take a moment and think about all the people you make sacrifices for. Now think about how many of them make sacrifices for you.

You probably tell yourself, or even that other person, that this is the last time you are going to help them, but eventually you help them again . . . and again, hoping that one day things will change. Hanging your hat on that kind of hope is insane, because insanity is doing the same thing over and over expecting to get different results. However, the day you stop making one-way sacrifices is the day you break the cycle of insanity.

I understand that you sometimes feel guilty

or see others putting their personal concerns in a locked box, and you don't want to appear that you are Selfish (1), but take a minute and think about all the women you know that put their personal concerns in a locked box. Are they healthy and happy and doing all the things they dream of? Probably not, so why continue to live that way if no one is happy?

That's what my mother calls being stuck on stupid. Just because everyone else is doing it that way does not mean you have to do it that way.

Ten O'clock: Example of Brain Surgery

Here's a story about how easy it is to perform a Brain Surgery to instantly change your thoughts and behavior.

In 1994, I was living in Houston, Texas, and I drove a Geo Tracker, which contained an automatic transmission, but I always wanted to learn how to drive a car with a manual transmission, or commonly referred to as driving a stick.

There was a week that my work assignment was in Galveston, Texas. One night, I stopped by a dealership to look at a Honda Civic.

I spoke to a salesman about what features I

wanted, which included a manual transmission. The next day, that salesman brought me a white Honda Civic with a stick on my lunch break.

By the way, earlier I mentioned I always wanted to drive a stick, but I didn't say that I knew how to drive one.

I asked him to drive it while I stayed in the passenger seat. I watched his feet and listened to the engine to mentally learn the concept of shifting gears. We concluded the test drive and 2 days later, I purchased that car and drove it home to Houston.

After driving an hour, I only stalled once two blocks away from my apartment. Pretty good for someone that never drove a stick before.

My point is that most things we do or don't do are because fear somehow holds our brain captive and we underestimate ourselves.

Imagine what your life would be like if you could only reprogram your mind to eliminate the fear and excuses, and then infect others with your wisdom to help them transform. Wow, keep that hope alive!

Tick Tock ⊘

CHAPTER 3

Application

. . . Apply your heart to instruction, and your ears to the words of knowledge (Proverbs 23:12).

In the Introduction (Rise & Shine), I referenced the phrase *knowledge is power,* and that I learned from motivational speaker Jonathan Sprinkles that knowledge isn't power at all, but that *applied* knowledge is power. I walked away from his presentation realizing that knowledge is merely information taking up space in my brain, and it's dormant until I actually do something with it.

My brain needed to CTRL+ALT+DEL after his presentation because I was conditioned for years to read as much as I could and to know a little about a lot of things. That day was another turning point in my pursuit to becoming a female masterpiece.

Here's a simple example of applied knowledge. Imagine that you're sitting in a restaurant and someone begins to choke on their food, but you don't help that person. Yet, 2 months prior, you learned in a safety class how to apply the Heimlich maneuver.

In this example, you have the knowledge to save the person from passing out or dying, but you didn't apply that invaluable knowledge. You see, you can know a lot about many things, but if you don't know when to use that knowledge, it's just worthless information marinating in your head and taking up space.

Now that you know about Vision and Brain Surgery, let's move on to the last key element to maximizing your time and being happy while you do it.

Eleven O'clock: Get It Done

The final part of 24 is dedicated to providing you with tips on how you can get things done without getting outdone. As I previously mentioned under Rise & Shine, I call them: Time Efficiency Tips™ (TETs). TETs are easy, everyday things you can do to conquer the things you want or need to do without creating excuses.

Excuses are crutches we use to make ourselves

feel better or to justify why we aren't committed to the Vision. I love the way an Unknown Author defines excuses: "Excuses are the tools of the weak and incompetent used to build monuments of nothingness. Those who excel in it seldom excel in anything else but excuses." Ouch!

Now, when it comes to conquering a *To Do* List, I am the queen conqueror. Carol, one of my closest friends, laughs at me all the time because she marvels over how I can get 10–15 things checked off my list in 1 day.

When I set out to shop or run errands, I don't get distracted and I don't bring distractions with me.

To be honest, I don't like shopping with other people, and I never go "window-shopping." It's a waste of time for me and slows me down. I shop online for 90 percent of my clothing and shoes. That's just me, but try going shopping alone 1 day and see just how much you can get done. I guarantee you'll notice a big difference in how much time you save and how much you accomplish.

While writing this book, I developed a support network titled "Living Life Without Excuses" group. This group consisted of women who were mothers, wives, single parents, teachers, retirees . . . just plain ordinary folks.

Every morning around 5:30, I texted them with a suggested workout plan for the day, a motivational push, or a simple reminder to stay focused. The workouts were quick and easy to execute throughout the day. Yes, I said *throughout the day*!

Here are examples of the texts:

Start with 60 crunches, then raise your leg like a dog at a fire hydrant and swing your leg parallel to the ground while brushing your teeth. Tighten the abs and booty. Do a minute on each leg.

In the shower or on the "porcelain": Do one set of 15 triceps.

Do not eat any sweets today.

On Saturdays, I texted a challenge to the group to see how many of whatever exercise I named that each lady could do within the course of a day. That night, the ladies who participated would send me a text reply stating how many they did.

Throughout the course of the month, I texted the ladies pictures and tips on sugar-free snacks, protein drinks, low-sugar juices, and supplements that I tried and that tasted pretty good.

Many ladies began calling me while they were grocery shopping as a means to putting healthy food and snacks in their shopping carts. It was helpful for them to know that somebody else had tried different products so that they didn't waste time and money.

I experimented with the group for about a year and a half and the feedback I received was overwhelmingly positive. Most of the ladies insisted that my method was inspiring and challenging and that they achieved desired results.

Twelve O'clock: Time Efficiency Tips™ (TETs)

The next few pages are dedicated to providing you numerous TETs. These TETs are radical and extreme for people who really want to change their life, get things done, and more importantly, see results. I've done all of these TETs at some point in my adult life, and many of them I still do every day.

The listing is in no specific or logical order. When you read them, you'll first say to yourself that Dana Simone Stovall is crazy, but the truth is I'm fanatical about maintaining control of my life and the happiness therein—without excuses. And I want that for you too!

Time Efficiency Tips™

1. Mirror Graffiti Reminders

Use lipstick to write personal notes on the bathroom mirror. You probably spend a great deal of time standing in front of it, at least 30 minutes throughout the day, so while you're standing there brushing your teeth and combing your hair, you can program your mind with the things you need to focus on for the day. The more you see something in writing, the more inclined you are to remember it. At this moment, my mirror reflects: Stay focused! Write something on your mirror right now.

2. Closet Psychology

For my readers that are trying to lose weight, avoid buying clothes to accommodate your current size, but buy clothes in the size you want to be. If you continue to buy clothes that fit your current size, what's the motivation to lose the weight? Exactly! There is none.

Get several outfits in the size you desire to fit into and hang them on your bedroom door or somewhere visible in your house. The clothes become an incentive to work out and stay focused for at least two reasons: because you really want to be that size and because you're pissed off that you spent money on clothes you can't even wear yet. Now if that's not motivation, I don't know what is.

Many of you may say that's a waste of money to buy clothes you can't fit into. What's the difference between the clothes hanging on your door that you can't wear and the clothes of numerous sizes in your closet that you can't fit into? Hmmm . . . Moving on.

3. Moonlight Dictation

If you're like me, I tend to brainstorm in the middle of the night. Keep a handheld recorder or a pad and pencil next to your bed to quickly jot down those thoughts. Then when you wake up in the morning, put it in your planner or on your mirror. This ensures that you don't forget those o'dark 30 brain surges.

4. Staircase Delivery

Have you ever taken note of how many times you go up and down the stairs because you forgot to get something or to take something up or down?

Put things at the top or bottom of your stairs to remind you (or others) to deliver it to its respective location. For example, clothes from the laundry or shoes that have made a mountain at the front door. I also put Destiny's school notes that require my signature at the top of the stairs so she remembers to grab them on her way to the bus stop.

5. Children: Homework = Mom: Workout

While your children are completing their homework, get a workout in. They don't need you to walk through their assignment every day, they need you to check it and explain their errors when they're done. You think that you are helping them when you walk them through it, but really, you are wasting time. Remember, typically they spent the day learning the concept of their assignment. The homework is merely to reinforce it. Even if it only takes them 5 minutes or 30, any amount of time you spend exercising is more beneficial than expending no time at all.

6. Head-to-Toe Packing

Don't you hate when you travel somewhere

only to find out when you get there that you forgot something? I've created a solution for that problem. While you are packing, touch every body part to ensure that whatever item related to that respective body part gets packed. For example, when I touch my feet, I think of shoes, socks, toenail polish, flip-flops, pumice bar, ankle bracelet, and toe ring. Or when I touch my hair, I think of rollers, satin bonnet, gel, holding spray, bobby pins, pony-tail holders, shampoo/conditioner, oil sheen, and a sun hat.

Once you know the things you need for each body part, packing becomes easy, and forgetting to pack something is unlikely.

7. Baby Onboard

As a new mom, we are inclined to feel guilty when we can't hold our babies when they want you to because we need to wash dishes or do other household chores. Here's a hands-free tip that I learned from one of my African au pairs that I did all the time with Destiny when she was a baby.

Take a piece of long, soft, durable fabric and

wrap it securely around your upper torso with your baby inside of it, similar to one of those heavier baby carriers. You can wrap your baby in front or on your back. This allows you to clean house or work out regularly without running back and forth to the nursery or constantly stopping what you're doing to play with the baby.

Your little bundle will love being close to you all the time and listening to your heartbeat. As a matter of fact, nap times became generally effortless.

Additionally, it's really fun for your baby if you lay on your back and secure them to your chest, and do sit-ups because as you properly breathe through the movement, exhale in your baby's face and they will think it's a game.

8. Color Tracking

Many people look at my day planner and they say, "What the heck?!" because many of my entries are highlighted in different colors. I highlight bills that are due in blue, my paydays in green, and my days off/holidays in pink.

Our brains are like computers. Once we program them, they will apply that function anytime we want. For example, as you know, the colors of the traffic light represent a different command: stop (red), prepare to stop or proceed with caution (yellow), and go (green). Those three colors are merely global functions that our brains respond to no matter where we go or what we are doing.

I apply that same concept to my daily planner to stay organized to get things done and done timely. When I see a green entry, my mind begins to process the fact that I need to do my weekly budget. When I see a blue entry, I ask myself, has payment been made already through my online bill payment software or is there an automatic electronic funds transfer (EFT) set up with that creditor or company.

I've had this color-coded system in place since my 20s. My bills are rarely late, and as a result, my credit score is over 700. Develop your own color tracking to stay ahead of the game.

9. Mobile Phone Automation

Did you know that your cell phone has reminder and calendar functions? Try using them in addition to or instead of your planner. Your phone is more likely to be with you at all times than your planner anyway. I use the reminders for everything because I admit, I forget things unless I write them down.

Many phones allow you to schedule the reminder for a certain day and time as well as provide you with a reminder an hour or 2 before the actual time.

You can remind yourself to run an errand, pick up milk, exercise, watch *Scandal*, pay bills, schedule doctor appointments, and return phone calls. Whatever you need to remember, set up a reminder. If it has to be done, my phone calendar knows more about it than I do.

10. Crave Control

How many times do you get a craving for a little snack but the only thing in your reach is that cookie bouquet or the bowl of M&Ms at the receptionist desk? The way to control what you eat during a craving is to stay armed with healthy snacks in your purse, desk, and car. This is especially necessary when you go grocery shopping. More times than not, we find ourselves buying groceries when we're hungry and inevitably the shopping cart becomes full of carbs, trans fat, and sodium.

It's also a good idea to keep healthy snacks on hand because in the event of an unexpected traffic delay, car failure, or an extremely long office meeting, your first thought is to grab something quick (fast food) on the way home. So instead, grab something healthy from your purse.

11. Time Allocation

Just like many of you prepare a budget by alloting a portion of your income to your expenses, the same concept should be applied to preparing your *To Do* List.

Next to each task, you should write down the estimated amount of time it normally takes you to complete it, including travel time to and from and a 5-minute cushion for the unexpected (e.g., pick up dry cleaning—20 minutes). If you have six hours available on Saturday to complete your tasks, then the aggregate minutes on your *To Do* List should not exceed six hours.

In addition, make sure you leave your list on the refrigerator and discuss it with your spouse and children in the event you missed a ballet practice or something and the list needs to be revised accordingly. More importantly, the list should be discussed with others so that they are aware of what you intend to accomplish that day.

The more you consistently stick to your list, the less likely your spouse or children will feel inclined to hijack it.

12. I'm on a Diet . . . Starting Monday

One of the things that people say that makes me want to scream is "On Monday, I'm starting my diet." I then say to myself, *and how many Mondays this year have you started a diet?*

While it's realistic to set a target date for buying a house or car or planting a garden, it's never a good idea to set a date to start a diet. Once you've gone through Brain Surgery and decided to lose weight, the moment you start to make that change is at that very moment. If you allow yourself to set a diet date, that date will always be a moving target in your mind. As a result, if you fall off the wagon, all you do is choose another date to start. This is the main reason why you don't see results, so do yourself a favor and stop cheating.

13. The Restaurant Trap

Another reason why people overeat is because many restaurants "overserve." But guess what? You don't have to eat it all.

As soon as the waiter brings your meal, immediately ask for a carryout container. Don't touch any of it until you put half of the meal in the box. Once you see what's left on your plate, your brain sends a signal to your stomach indicating that this portion is going to fill you up. And psychologically, it does. After you eat the smaller portion, you won't feel stuffed or miserable, just satisfied. Try it; it works every time.

14. Dinnertime Child Abuse

Similar to the premise of TET 13, refrain from preparing a large plate of food for your children, and telling them to eat everything on their plate... or else.

Although kids are growing, we as parents have to regulate their portions and their physical activities accordingly. Put smaller portions on their plate and let them ask for more. Then give them a little more, but not a portion larger than the first plate.

Unless you have a very active child (that plays sports or aggressively plays outside daily), giving them large meal portions can lead to obesity and severe self-esteem issues. By the way, a child that sits in the house watching TV and playing video games for hours is *not* classified as being physically active.

As a matter of fact, there may come a time when you will have to take away the video games in order to motivate your children to become more physically active. I decided a long time ago that video games and the TV would not be used more than the vacuum cleaner or the treadmill in my house.

If your child is already showing signs of excessive weight, nip their eating habits in the bud right now. Stop trying to convince yourself that he or she will "grow out of it" because they probably won't.

As a parent, it is your responsibility to foster a healthy lifestyle for your children. You may not be able to control your own eating habits, but remember, you still control your children's habits as long as they live in your house.

15. Location, Location, Location

Where is the worst place to put your treadmill and other workout equipment? The Basement!! Unless you go into the basement frequently throughout the day, it doesn't belong there. Why?

Out of sight, out of mind.

Location isn't just the key rule to real estate, it's also the key rule for workout equipment for home use. When the equipment is conveniently located, you are more likely to use it, even if the equipment doesn't look appealing in an area that you spend most of your time in.

It's not about the equipment looking good, it's about the equipment helping *you* look good.

16. Let It Ring—Turn It Off

The telephone and TV are other habits that eat into your use of time. When you are busy running errands and other *To Do* tasks, don't answer the phone. Send the caller into voice mail. If it's important, they'll leave a message;

otherwise, it's not worth the distraction. Walking around trying to hold a conversation and get things done does not work well at all because it slows you down.

Ladies, turn off the TV. It's such a distraction. If you need noise while you're cleaning or cooking or whatever, listen to some music. Listening to music doesn't distract some people as much as the TV. As a matter of fact, music helps your efficiency because of the flow you create instinctively from the rhythm of the music.

I keep my TV off so much that I forget to turn it on sometimes.

17. Drink Up

For many of us, drinking the right amount of water daily can be a challenge. The reason I dislike drinking water so much is because I don't like stopping in the middle of doing something to go tinkle. Pray, church!

So here's a good TET: put a bottle with frozen water in your bathroom at night. In the morning, the ice is almost melted so while getting dressed, drink the entire bottle before heading downstairs to leave for work. Before you walk out the door, grab another bottle of water from the refrigerator, then drink it in the car or on the train on the way to work or your destination. Before noon, drink another bottle, then on your way home from work or wherever, drink another bottle before you've reached your destination.

By doing this, before you arrive home for the evening, you will have eight glasses of water in your system.

18. The Refrigerator Is the Devil

People that have seen the inside of my refrigerator sometimes say that I need to go grocery shopping. I tell them that I don't. My refrigerator has everything that Destiny and I need to consume per week. Just because the refrigerator is 6 feet tall doesn't mean that I need 6 feet of food in it. Having a full refrigerator is not always a good thing, especially when it's filled with crappy food.

If you are trying to maintain a healthy lifestyle, the inside of your refrigerator should look healthy.

Some women tell me that their husbands and

children don't want to eat that healthy. Guess what, ladies? Let them know that they won't eat or they can go out to dinner without you. Don't make a separate meal for them and don't buy the junk food that they like. None of it belongs in the house, because you don't need the temptation to choose a different diet date.

I'm not saying cook tofu or rice cake casserole every day for dinner, but you should be able to prepare healthy meals that you and the family will enjoy without compromising your health and fitness.

19. Create a Habit

I learned during a women's health and fitness retreat from Dawn Jackson Blatner, the founder of the Flexitarian Diet, that you have to first create a habit before you can put in the effort to accomplish a goal. For example, if you want to start going to the gym, Dawn suggested that you get dressed and just drive to the gym and don't do anything when you get there for 1 whole week. That creates the habit of going to the gym. Then after 1 week, begin to do a few exercises and build the intensity week after week.

It may sound silly, but when she said this, I immediately thought to myself, what a great form of Brain Surgery.

20. Football or Cheer Practice Is YOUR Time

When you take your children to their activities, don't just sit there chatting with the other moms. Go get a massage, a manicure, or even better, do some squats, lunges, or use the dumbbells in your car (hint, hint). It's called double-dipping. They do what they have to do, and you do what you need to do simultaneously. It's like Hannah Montana, the best of both worlds.

21. Sunday Cook-A-Thon

If you are anything like me, I do not like cooking when I get home from work every day. Not to mention that if your children or your spouse is home before you, they could have already prepared dinner, but I won't go there.

Here's a good tip: on Sundays, prepare your dinner for the whole week. No need to get fancy. Things such as spaghetti, soup, baked or fried chicken, rice dishes, short ribs, casseroles, or chili are perfect. Label each pan Monday, Tuesday, Wednesday, etc., so everyone knows what the dinner plans are for each evening.

Prepare the salad or steam any complementing veggies when you get home; or better yet, leave a note for the family advising them to steam the broccoli or fix the salad before you arrive home. Since everyone wants to eat, everyone needs to pitch in.

My absolute favorite is meals prepared in a Crock-Pot. You just throw the ingredients in before bedtime and it's done before you leave for work in the morning. Don't stress yourself out over dinner. It's supposed to be the smallest meal of the day anyway. You can ask me why in an email after you read this book.

Exercise Opportunities: Morning, Noon, and Night

The next three TETs are my favorite! Remember under Rise & Shine, I stated that I would show you how to exercise at least three times a day? After you read TETs 22-24, I'll bet you a bag of Hot Fries that there are at least three workout opportunities that you can begin doing today.

Ladies, before you begin exercising regularly, speak with a trainer or an experienced person on proper techniques to execute your exercises. If you ever wonder why you aren't seeing better results from your exercise plan, it's probably due to improper execution. Every exercise you do is intended to concentrate on one or more muscles. In addition, there's a posture, breathing, and muscle contraction that should be applied.

22. Fitness on Wheels

When you think of exercising, what place comes to mind? You immediately thought of a fitness center, right? The problem with the gym is that most of the people reading this book will say that they don't have time for that.

You see, for most women, it takes energy and

planning to GO somewhere to exercise. So I have the perfect excuse-buster plan.

First, purchase a set of ankle and wrist weights and a set of 3-, 5-, or 8-pound dumbbell weights. Next, put a set of the dumbbells in your car, your office/cubicle, next to the sofa or chair you sit in while watching TV, in the carpool vehicle, and in the two bathrooms you use the most at home.

In the car, at the red lights, grab your dumbbells and do chest presses, shoulder presses, or triceps and biceps curls until the light changes. This is also great for people who sit in traffic daily or have long commutes to work. People stare at me like I'm crazy, but guess what? I bet they wish they had a set of dumbbells in their car too.

23. WWW: Working Out While Working

One of my favorite times to exercise is at the office during listen-only conference calls. Just put your phone on speaker and mute, raise the volume, and hit the floor and do abdominal exercises during the entire call. Don't forget your dumbbells. You can even add a 90-degree wall squat.

24. Exhaust All the Possibilities

There is nothing you do or no place you go that should prohibit you from getting a little exercise. While shopping, running errands, or taking the commuter train, put your leg or wrist weights on. While brushing your teeth, stirring a pot, or even washing dishes, do squats, lunges, donkey kicks, or side leg extensions.

I'm sure you're saying to yourself right now "wow, that's crazy!" And you're right, it is. But I like to refer to it as *fanatical fitness*.

So, how many potential workout moments did I suggest? And none of these exercises required more of your time at all. They merely *maximize* the time you already have.

By the way, I'll be expecting my bag of Hot Fries within the week.

Tick Tock ☺

Nightcap

Phew! Are you excited or just exhausted thinking about where to go from here? That's the beauty of this book. You don't have to stress out or get outdone to make the decision to get your life back on track. You already have the Vision, the Brain Surgery is scheduled, now all you have to do is submit to the Application.

I'm not naïve to think that all of you will agree with my philosophy. My approach is definitely radical and not the normal advice you would receive from your therapist, religious advisor, doctor, or personal trainer, but take a look at your current normal. Is it working? Are you honestly happy? I'm just saying . . .

Now, men, I know many of you will read this book too. The woman in your life needs your help with her transformation. It will be hard adjusting to being a big boy, taking care of yourself more often, and relying less on her to micromanage your grown behind. But in the long run, you too will benefit from her new normal. Remember that quote, "If momma ain't happy, ain't nobody happy." Lighten up a little and give her a break. She deserves your unconditional support. Besides, isn't it better to support her while she lives with you, then for her to find a different zip code and be supported by someone else? Sorry! I'm just pointing out one of those blind spots.

There's nothing holding you back.

You can only play the game of life once, so make your own rules and play it the way you want to. I'm confident that you will be happier and healthier, emotionally and physically.

Say good-bye to fear forever.

Warn your family and friends that you are having Brain Surgery and that they should brace themselves for your "new normal."

Demolish the walls of your comfort zone.

Change is never comfortable. That's why many people resist and avoid it by any means necessary. Today, I ask you to think of your change as mandatory, and consider it from a different perspective. We all know, there are three stages within the life cycle of a butterfly: caterpillar, to pupa/chrysalis, to butterfly. There is nothing comfortable about a caterpillar being suffocated by leaves into a mummy-like structure hanging from a branch like a bat for an extended period of time. But when that butterfly breaks out of the pupa, it's one of nature's most beautiful creatures. So when you want to complain during your metamorphosis about being uncomfortable, just think about how beautiful and empowered you will look and feel when you break out of your shell.

I pray wholeheartedly that you enjoyed reading 24 as much as I enjoyed writing it.

I'll grab the cape--then meet me at the phone booth!

Zzz